How to Conquer Gout?

Teresa Szabo

How to Conquer Gout?

Teresa Szabo

Published by LULU
San Diego, California 2010

Title
How to Conquer Gout

Author
Teresa Szabo

Cover Design
Marcin Kubik

Translation from Polish
Marcin Kubik

Editor
Marcin Kubik

Published by LULU 2010

ISBN 978-0-557-72321-8

TABLE OF CONTENTS

Introduction

My purpose in writing this book is to convince people suffering from pain caused by gout, of the possibility of aid.

Only through proper diet, avoidance of purine rich foods, drinking plenty of water, getting at least 6 to 8 hours of sleep and through elimination of constipation, I was finally able to return to full health.

The process of my return to complete health lasted well over two years.

After reading this book, application of the methods presented and rigorous adherence to the gout diet, you will be able to reduce your return to complete health to several weeks.

Recipes presented in the last chapter, very tasty and easy to prepare, are the basis to completely free you from the pain caused by gout.

I note that the modern conventional medicine does not have a thorough knowledge, nor does it offer any effective cure for gout. The lack of doctors specializing in the treatment of this disease is a major hurdle in the process of recovery.

Medications used to treat gout are made from synthetic chemicals and produce a wide variety of side effects.

Other methods used by me in the fight against gout include learning to breathe properly, developing and making a habit of „the morning ritual" and sound discipline in the application of diet.

The behavioral system developed and presented in this book will greatly help the reader understand the needs of the human organism and gout. As a result, it will allow him to return to a life free of fear that the next attack of pain is imminent.

Development of a new habit <u>requires only thirty days</u>.

It is wroth the effort to free yourself of sleepless nights, days missed at work and the associated financial loss, tense atmosphere at home, forever lost days spent in pain, deformed joints, and the prospect of faster death. The effort is definitely worth it.

I wish you pleasant reading and a life without further gout attacks.

Teresa Szabo

Preface

Dear Reader!

The book you hold in your hands will clarify all the reasons why you developed gout. Thanks to this book you will free yourself of gout and all its effects: tragic, systematic attacks of excruciating pain.

After years of observation and experiencing progressively increasing in strength attacks of pain, after countless hours spent on the web sites devoted to health and disease, after reading many, many books on these subjects I finally understood the complex causes of my illness, gout.

I designed a diet, which has helped me in ridding my body of old uric acid deposits. The presented diet comes with ready recipes for the proper nutrition of a gout sufferer. And that's not all!

I present „golden rules", for instance: never eat almonds and nuts alone by themselves, which are very nutritious, but must <u>exclusively</u> be eaten with brown rice.

You will find explanations of the workings of your digestive system, with a special emphasis on friendly bacteria, without which we, gout sufferers, are unable to properly and effectively, excrete the excess of uric acid. I present information detailing natural sources, thanks to which you can rebuild your bacterial flora.

I developed and explained the water drinking method – why it is so important in your metabolic process. You will also get an explanation as to why you should only drink filtered or mineral water.

In this book you will find a priceless method of the morning routine, which will teach you what to do in the first 90 minutes after awakening. The effects resulting from this method are priceless; they cannot be converted to any sum of money.

After getting to know the breathing method and its practical use, you will quickly make progress in getting the right amount of oxygen into your body, which will greatly speed up your recovery process.

Dear Reader, upon having studied and gained an understanding of the causes of why you developed gout, you will easily apply your new knowledge and free yourself from gout once and for all – just as I have done.

I wish you speedy recovery.

Teresa Szabo

Definitions of Gout

After being diagnosed with gout, I began my search for information regarding this illness on the Internet. I developed my own definition of gout, since the material I have researched was inconsistent, even in the naming of the disease itself.

The reasons for gout were always the same: excess production of uric acid and problems with its removal from the body.

Gout is an illness resulting from excess uric acid in the human body, which is not properly removed by the excretory and digestive systems, undergoing the process of crystallization. Usually it crystallizes in joints, at the ends of bones and in muscles. This process causes excruciating, ripping pain and the areas infected with the acid swell considerably.

Gout can be sometimes confused with pseudo gout (Chondrocalcinosis).

It is my belief that both of those ailments have their roots in improper **diet**.

Pseudo gout is a form of join inflammation that occurs due to the accumulation of a specific type of calcium crystals.

Since, over time, more and more crystals are deposited in the joints, they can cause reactions that lead to severe pain and swelling. Swelling may be short-term or long-term and occurs most often in the knees, but may also occur in the wrists, arms, ankles or hands.

The pain caused by pseudo gout is sometimes so excruciating that a person may be prevented from performing normal daily life functions for many days.

As the name itself suggests, pseudo gout's symptoms are similar to those caused by primary gout.

Pseudo gout may resemble rheumatoid arthritis or degenerative joint disease. A correct diagnosis is essential because untreated it can lead to arthritis and joint deformation.

Pseudo gout most often affects the elderly, occurring in approximately 3% of people over 60 years of age and up to 50% of people over 90 years old.

Causes of pseudo gout.

The causes of this disease are unknown. It is known however that the risk increases

significantly with age, hence it is possible that the physical and chemical changes that accompany aging increase susceptibility to pseudo gout.
Other diseases, both former and present may also have an impact on gout susceptibility. These include: hypothyroidism, genetic disorder of iron overload (hemochromatosis) or elevated calcium level in blood (hypercalcemia).

Pseudo gout can also be caused by damage to joints, resultant for instance from trauma or surgery, or it can be result of stress from another disease.

If the causes of pseudo gout are identified and treated, it is possible to prevent future attacks.

Very often, however, there are no identified causes for this disease and in such cases there is no way to prevent recurring attacks of pseudo gout from happening.

Gout is a rich man's disease - as someone once called it - and has been known for centuries.

Why a rich man's disease?

In the past only the rich could afford to put a lot of meat, fats and alcohol on their tables.

The attack cycle

I have observed my gout attacks for over a year, to get an understanding of how and exactly when they begin.

Meticulously made notes in a thick book have helped me in examining the complex factors that could affect the next gout attack.

I wrote down all the food products used in my menu, the amount of water I consumed, how I felt after the meal, and what I experienced during the day. I made note of the number of defecations or their absence.

I finally understood that the reason behind the attack is simply uric acid poisoning. Symptoms are the same as in other poisoning instances.

I felt chills, my nervousness increased; I was irritated and edgy for no good reason. I became quarrelsome, intolerant and not understanding of myself and others.

Fatigue and sleeplessness, are the first signs of a coming attack. Slowed reflexes, a feeling of breathlessness and anxiety grow hour by hour. The cause of all these ill feelings is in reality the result of one factor – uric acid poisoning.

The body begins to fight back and the immune system tries to take control of the situation, aiming to preserve the delicate balance of all the processes constantly carried on in our organism.

Sometimes the attack was weak and passed quickly. Then it left behind „beat up places" – where the acid has crystallized and deposited. When pressed, such areas would produce pain just like a bruise caused by a hit or injury. The locations were various. They appeared under the eyes, on top of the skull, in hands, arms, palms, fingers, basically everywhere. Sometimes they invaded several places at once.

The „beat up places" came to my attention much earlier, years before the emergence of intensive and very painful attacks.

With the strong attacks, the cycle duration has increased to several days and sometimes up to a few weeks. The onset of the attack was exhibited by lack of comfort, short and restless sleep, increased appetite, and nervousness.

Everything started to irritate me. Nothing made me happy. I experienced temporary attacks of depression.

The duties of everyday life did not always allow me to notice the early symptoms and thus made me incapable of reacting to them in any way –

not even by a simple method like drinking an increased amount of warm water with lemon.

During the main phase of the attack, when the excess acid accumulated, in places where the body would find room for it and the crystallization process began, there appeared a disgusting, severe, ripping pain.

These very long hard needles of acid crystals, exert pressure on soft tissues of the bones, tendons and muscles, causing a pain so unbearable that one doesn't know where or how to hide from it.

The duration of such an attack varies widely. It depends on the "infraction" committed in the diet, and any deviation from regular consumption of sufficient quantities and the amount of proper rest. It is also dependent on other ailments – a runny nose or common cold – both a can go hand in hand with acid overproduction.

Severe soreness in the muscles after physical exercise or strenuous physical effort can also trigger a gout attack.

The lactic acid produced in the muscles causes an additional burden on the immune system, delaying the expulsion of the excess uric acid.

Our immune system if it is busy with fighting off other enemies – bacteria, viruses, or any of various other microorganisms, unknown in the body until the moment of invasion, begins to treat <u>excess</u> uric acid removal as a matter of secondary importance. In other words it starts to "pack" the acid into whatever free space it finds available, storing it for later removal.

During the crystallization of the uric acid the affected area reddens itches and swells significantly.

The swelling persists for several days and sometimes several weeks. It completely depends on the overall health condition of the body. For example, during something as simple as a common cold, the swelling can persist even for a few weeks.

A swollen knee, wrist or hand strongly inhibits free movement. Sometimes I stumbled about on a swollen, painful leg for three or four weeks.

If an acid infection occurred in my arms, I wasn't able to sleep because I couldn't find a comfortable position to lie in. In such moments, I could only nap in a sitting position.

Getting some good rest during gout attacks is truly a very difficult task and takes lots of time and concentration.

Medications

In general, one must be extremely careful and personally responsible in the use of drugs to treat an illness or ailment.

Worth remembering: all drugs synthetically created in pharmaceutical factories, produced chemically from a variety of components, have side effects that affect other organs. Those effects are often irreversible, sometimes causing permanent disability or even death.

The manufacturers of drugs are primarily interested in achieving big profit margins from their production, and perhaps less interested in the well being of the patient.

Even though the United States and Europe do have special agencies responsible for regulating and supervising the production and effectiveness of each medication, which are sold exclusively under professional medical supervision (prescription drugs), one has to be very cautious in taking drugs and carefully follow the instructions of the doctor who has prescribed them.

In addition, I recommend that before using any type of medication prescribed, its effectiveness is discussed with the doctor and questions regarding any potential side effects are freely asked and thoroughly clarified.

Caution against the use of drugs without a prescription should be even stronger. Complete absence of control over the drug raises questions about its effectiveness and its potential side effects.

In the specific case of gout, the pharmacological market has several drugs available for the gout sufferer.

Personally I did not use any of them, since their side effects are too numerous and too dangerous.

Allopurinol (Zyloprim) (a prescription drug) inhibits uric acid synthesis and has been linked to skin eruptions, inflammation of the blood vessels, and liver toxicity.

Periodic liver enzymes, renal function tests and complete blood counts should be performed in all patients on allopurinol.

Alterations in liver enzymes, including transient elevations of serum alkaline phosphatase, AST and ALT, have occurred in some patients.

Reversible hepatomegaly, hepatocellular damage (including necrosis), granulomatous changes, hepatitis and jaundice have also occurred.

Colchicine (a prescription drug) is used to alleviate attacks. This drug can cause serious side effects and toxicity and even death in high doses.

Side Effects: 80% of people, who take colchicine in doses that are high enough to be effective, develop stomach problems such as cramping, nausea, diarrhea, or vomiting.

Serious side effects of colchicine include bone marrow problems, muscle inflammation, severe anemia, and extremely low white blood counts that can increase the risk of infection developing.

Colchicine is usually avoided or the dose adjusted in people who have reduced kidney function.

Indomethacin is a non-steroidal anti-inflammatory drug (NSAID). NSAID's have become the treatment of choice among doctors and Indomethacin is the most widely used prescription drug for most gout attacks.

NSAID's may also have significant toxicity, but if used for the SHORT TERM they are generally well tolerated.

Prednisone is being prescribed for gout more and more these days. This immunosuppressive drug, though necessary in some cases, is associated with serious long-term side effects such as cataracts, bone loss, weakening of the immune system, and many others.

One of the most serious complications from prednisone is the risk of osteoporosis, which occurs from the bone loss.

The most commonly reported side effects are increased acid in the stomach, sodium retention, delayed healing, decreased ability to fight infection, bone and muscle problems, acne, night sweats, increased sugar in the blood, and thrush (yeast growth in the mouth which is a very strong indication of the lack of "friendly" bacteria in the body- resources strongly needed to fight infection).

As with many other medications, Prednisone will cover up the disease but it is the underlying problem, the cause of the disease, which must be repaired.

Pain relief

In general, I appreciate the scientific achievements of modern medicine. What concerns me, however, is why so little scientific research is done to remove the causes of gout, and in effect, to prevent the incredible pain that accompanies it.

In practice, the available pharmacological means for gout pain are ineffective.

While it is true that painkillers reduce suffering during a gout attack, the side effects of a synthetically produced pill usually cause the uric-acid to re-deposit and consequently create the next attack.

The reader may consider it cruel, but I strongly advise against taking any painkillers at all. Not even Ibuprofen.

All synthetic drugs, including the popular aspirin, lay a heavy burden on the liver and form acids, which delay the removal of uric acid from the body.

What methods did I use during gout attacks in order to reduce pain? Here they are:

Cold compresses on the sore spots, they bring relief and more. Cold helps remove the acid from sore places and inhibits crystallization – the formation of long, hard needles of crystal.

I used different methods for cold compresses. Sometimes I simply wrapped a few ice cubes in a small towel and held it to the sore spot. Other times I purchased cold therapy products which also served to reduce pain.

Warm compresses I applied after first using the cold therapy. The heat warmed painful areas and helped blood circulation in the infected spot. The free inflow of blood facilitated the removal of uric acid.

Drinking warm water with lemon during attacks of pain; I often drank warm water with several drops of fresh lemon juice. It's a very effective method. On some occasions, I drank two to three quarts of water within a few hours. The warm water stimulated the liver and kidneys to function better and steady removal of toxins took place, including the removal of uric acid.

Tiger balm - traditionally it used to include powdered tiger bone but it now consists of purely herbal ingredients. I used this traditional Chinese medicine to heat rub areas of pain and wrapped them with a scarf, a towel, or put on a warm sock. If the joint affected was a knee or an elbow, I cut an opening "at the toes" of the sock and pulled it over the ailing knee, elbow or ankle. The balm heated and reduced pain, the sock protected bed sheets and clothing from dirtying.

Shower - I often took showers during the attacks. I changed water temperature, from cold to warm and hot. The water cleared the toxins and simultaneously massaged my body. The effect was immediate, and pain was reduced. The shower increased blood circulation, which in turn helped to clear the affected area from acid excess.

An interesting fact: 70% of the toxins removed by the body are removed through the skin.

I also used to alternate temperatures in the shower, from cold to warm and hot.
These showers brought excellent pain relief.

Physical activity - especially during the attacks I made an effort to be more physically active. Walking, twitching, waving of arms helped to "calm" the unbearable pain. When moving, circulation improved and the process of acid crystallization was markedly slowed, giving my organism a chance to excrete the excess uric acid.

Friendly Bacteria (Probiotics)

In my opinion, one of the basic conditions required is the elimination of constipation. Defecation must be regular, daily, or even twice a day. It should come naturally, with no great effort, and the feces should have soft consistency.

It is a very important condition that must be met in order to regain full Health.

Regular defecation is entirely dependent on the bacterial flora in the digestive system, and the intestines in particular. This is exactly what the friendly bacteria help to do, and that's the reason why I'm writing about them in greater detail.

If dear reader, you take a trip to the supermarket or look through various Health related articles in magazines and internet websites, chances are you will encounter Friendly Bacteria products, in capsule form, powdered, or other.

I have used friendly bacteria in capsule form for several weeks. In combination with my gout diet, I was easily able to rebuild by bacterial flora and all sings of constipation have disappeared, while pain attacks were more sporadic.

Just as a curiosity: from 1994 to 2003 Americans have tripled their expenditure for Friendly Bacteria and other supplements.

What are friendly bacteria?

One of the generally accepted definitions, created by the Food and Agriculture Organization of United Nations as well as the World Health Organization describes them as "Live microorganisms which when administered in adequate amounts confer a Health benefit on the host."

Microorganisms are tiny living organisms – such as bacteria, viruses and fungi – that can be seen only under a microscope.

Some of the conventional foods containing friendly bacteria are yogurt, fermented and unpasteurized milk, buttermilk, sour cream and Soya drinks.

In these foods, the bacteria may be originally present or be added during production. Most come from two groups of bacteria, Lactobacillus and Bifidobacterium. Within each group there are different species (e.g. Lactobacillus acidophilus and Bifidobacterium bifidus), and different strains (or varieties) are present within each individual species.

Scientific understanding of friendly bacteria and their potential for preventing and treating Health conditions is at an early stage, but it is consistently moving forward.

In November 2005, a conference was held by the American Society of Microbiologists in order to review the research results on the balance of bacterial flora in the human body.

Here is a brief summary of the topics discussed and conclusions reached during that conference.

Why are friendly bacteria (Probiotics) so important in human life?

The first encounter with the friendly bacteria takes places in infants shortly after birth. The world is full of microorganisms (including bacteria), and people have them on their skin, in their intestines and other organs.

Friendly bacteria are essential for the proper development of the immune system, for protection against factors that may cause illness, for the digestive process and for proper absorption of food and nutrients.

Bacterial flora is unique to the individual. The interactions between the person and the microorganisms in his or her body and the interactions between the microorganisms themselves can be crucial for that person's Health and wellbeing.

Imbalance in friendly bacteria (and other bacteria) may be caused by two main factors:

1. By antibiotics, which kill the friendly bacteria in the intestines along with the hostile infectious ones they're meant to eliminate.

2. Hostile microorganisms such as disease causing bacteria, yeast, fungi, parasites, can all upset the Probiotic balance.

Current friendly bacteria research entails several different areas. Scientists are trying to determine whether friendly bacteria can inhibit hostile bacterial growth and activity, in conditions such as:

- Diarrhea

- Irritable bowel syndrome

- Inflammatory bowel disease (e.g. ulcerative colitis and Crohn's disease)

- Bacterial infection by Helicobacter pylori (H. pylori), that usually causes ulcers and many types of chronic gastritis

- Tooth decay and gum disease

- Vaginal infections

- Stomach and respiratory infections

- Skin infections

According to a report from the conference, there is a persuasive body of evidence from studies of specific diseases, where friendly bacteria can be applied:

- In the treatment of diarrhea (especially diarrhea cause by rotavirus)

- In the prevention and treatment of viral infections in the reproductive system, urinary tract, and bacterial vaginosis

- In the treatment of irritable bowel syndrome

- To reduce the likelihood of urinary bladder cancer recurrence.

- To shorten the treatment process of intestinal infections caused by the bacteria Clostridium difficile.

- In order to prevent and manage atopic dermatitis (eczema) in children.

Friendly bacteria have traditionally been considered as useful in the treatment of various gastrointestinal diseases.

Uric acid (Urate)

Here is the definition of the acid as presented on the pages of Wikipedia:

Uric acid (2,6,8 Trioxypurine) is a purine derivative. Molecular formula: $C_5H_4O_3N_4$. It creates white crystals with low water solubility. At 400°C uric acid crystals decompose releasing hydrogen cyanide. It easily undergoes tautomerization.

Uricotelic organisms (such as birds, most reptiles, some insects and snails) excrete up to 90% of used up nitrogen in the form of uric acid. In mammals, small quantities of uric acid are present in the blood, liver, spleen, and urine. In humans and apes it is the end product of metabolized purines from digested food, de novo synthesis and degradation of endogenous nucleic acids.

Approximately 75% of uric acid is excreted in the urine, 25% goes to the gastrointestinal tract and is broken down by intestinal bacteria. The concentration of uric acid in healthy adults is 150-475 umol/L (2,5-8 mg/dl). Through urination an average of 500mg of uric acid is excreted daily either in free form or in the form of salt (depending on the pH of urine). Uric acid exhibits low water solubility and in an acid environment it

33

can accumulate in the joints and kidneys to form uric stones. In an alkaline environment it becomes easily soluble.

Uric acid is produced during the breakdown of purines, one of two classes of components of a complex of proteins and amino acids that make up DNA and RNA.

DNA – Deoxyribonucleic Acid – is a macromolecular organic compound belonging to the nucleic acids. It is found in the chromosomes and acts as a carrier of genetic information of living organisms.

RNA – Ribonucleic acid – is a molecule that consists of a long chain of nucleotide units, occurring in both the nucleus and in the cytoplasm of cells. There are many different classes of ribonucleic acids differing in both molecular weight and structure and responsible for a variety of functions.

Our bodies can process purines using the xanthine oxidase enzyme. But over-consumption of purine rich foods will produce more uric acid than the xanthine oxidase can handle.

Moreover, alcohol consumption, especially yeast containing beer, some diseases and drugs can weaken the enzyme system, so that the processing of normal levels of purines is disturbed. Any such imbalance can trigger an attack of gout pain.

In order to control the attacks of gout, one must control the uric acid concentration. <u>The first step</u> in controlling the uric acid concentration is the reduction in consumption of foods containing purines, because such foods increase uric acid production.

Alcohol has to avoided, because alcohol hinders renal function and accelerates the production of uric acid in the body.

It is also important to reduce the consumption of refined carbohydrates and saturated fats, avoid high protein diets, and consume amino acids which displace uric acid from the kidneys.

Excess uric acid produced due to reasons listed above, can deposit in muscle tissue and joints, over weeks, months or even years.

Once tissue is filled with uric acid, the crystallization of the acid takes place, which in turn causes the incredible pain of a gout attack.

Summing up all the causes of uric acid overproduction, one cannot forget such factors as:

- Renal failure
- Stress

- Alcohol consumption
- Vitamin deficiency
- Purine rich foods
- Illnesses, injuries, and surgeries undergone
- Medication taken without prescription
- Lack of friendly bacteria
- Obesity
- Antibiotics
- Cardiovascular problems
- All prescription drugs including those for gout
- Any joint damage
- Protein rich foods (such as meat, peas, beans, fish, crabs, shrimp, snails, etc.)
- Chlorinated water

Liver and kidneys are responsible for uric acid production. These same organs are also responsible for the removal of acid excess from the body.

It looks like a paradox, but this is how Mother Nature equipped us...

Chlorinated water

If you're not convinced of the dangers of chlorine in tap water, here is an extract of speech by an expert – Dr. Z. Ron.

"Most people do not think of chlorine as their great enemy. First of all, our elected officials carry on the propaganda guaranteeing that our chlorinated municipal water is completely safe for human consumption. Numerous scientific studies have reported that chlorinated water is a skin irritant and may be associated with rashes and blemishes. Chlorinated water can destroy polyunsaturated fatty acids and vitamin E in the body while generating toxins capable of free radical damage (oxidation). This may explain why supplementing one's diet with the necessary unsaturated fatty acids such as flax seed oil, evening primrose oil and borage as well as antioxidants such as vitamin E, selenium and others – help in many cases of eczema and dry skin conditions".

And further:

"Chlorinated water <u>destroys large part of the intestinal flora and friendly bacteria</u> that help digest food, which in turn protects the body from harmful pathogens.

These bacteria are responsible for the production of several important vitamins such as vitamin B12 and vitamin K. Chlorinated water is often the cause of chronic skin diseases such as acne, psoriasis, seborrhoeic dermatitis. To clean up or significantly improve skin conditions, chlorinated water should be changed to chlorine free water and add a dietary supplement with Lactobacillus acidophilus and friendly bacteria".

"Chlorinated water contains chemical compounds called trihalomethanes. They are carcinogenic agents resulting from a combination of chlorine and other compounds present in water. These chemicals, known as chlorinated hydrocarbons, are generally stored in fatty tissues of the body (breast, other fatty areas, mother's milk, blood and semen). Chlorinated hydrocarbons may cause DNA altering mutations, bypassing the immune system and interfering with natural control of cellular growth".

"Chlorine – this is documented – contributes to the worsening of asthma, especially in children who use chlorinated pools. A number of studies indicate that the effects of chlorine and chlorinated by-products contribute to higher incidence of inflammation of the bladder, breast and colorectal cancer, as well as malignant melanoma. One study has shown that the use of chlorinated water leads to congenital abnormalities of the heart. "

Anything you can do to filter tap and shower water to eliminate or at least minimize chlorine content, will undoubtedly be helpful and possibly curative for the immune system and may help eliminate several Health problems. The use of water filtration devices is becoming increasingly popular and cheaper. "If you have any questions or doubts on this subject – talk about it with your doctor".

Right after reading the above excerpt, I installed a tap water filter, even though I used water from my private well.

Breathing and relaxation

Breathing is one of the basic functions of our bodies, and all too often we fail to appreciate the importance of proper breathing for our Health.

The process of respiration is meant to provide "bubbles" of oxygen mainly to our brain, but also to all the other cells in our body, which thanks to oxygen can regenerate.

Oxygen is needed for the burning of carbon (chemical element). Carbon based organic compounds are continuously burned up by our bodies providing us with energy.

Some drink coffee or other "energy" drinks, to "revitalize and energize" the body. In fact, they are only deceiving themselves.

It is a matter of raising one's blood pressure which is caused by the secretion of adrenaline. When blood circulates faster, more oxygen gets to the cells at a faster rate.

This in turn allows for more "food" to be burned for energy and we feel "energized" while our well oxygenated brain feels more aware.

So when we learn to breathe properly or learn to control our blood pressure by proper breathing, we can liberate ourselves from all the side effects caused by caffeine.

Many religions and life philosophies have great respect for proper breathing. Numerous cultures believe that breathing is not only a purely chemical reaction, but a much more complex process of energy transfer, whose main "action" takes place at a metaphysical level.

When we learn to breathe properly (and therefore in conformity with nature, not as our civilization has forced upon us), we will be:

- Healthier
- We'll learn to control organs seemingly independent of human will like the heart, stomach, kidneys, liver (as well as blood pressure)
- We shall also gain advantages on a deeper spiritual level

Sometimes our bodies let us know that we need to take a deeper breath. This is why when we feel tired we tend to take deeper breaths by yawning.

And now for the practical part:

Hindu Yogis (master yoga practitioners who are specialists in proper breathing) distinguish three types of breathing:

1. Low breathing

2. Middle breathing
3. High breathing

And four phases of breath:

a. Inhalation
b. Pause after inhalation (full pause)
c. Exhalation
d. Pause after exhaling (empty pause)

1. Low breathing – this is the way men usually breathe. It mainly involves abdomen movement. The idea is to lower and expand the abdomen; by doing so we lower the diaphragm as low as possible and pull more air into the lungs. This is what low or diaphragm breathing looks like.

3. High breathing -   this is the way women usually breathe. It is breathing with your upper chest. We pull in our abdomen, the diaphragm goes up and we stick our chest out (to exaggerate to the movement we can bend back slightly and pull our shoulder blades together). We pull is as much air as possible!

2. Middle breathing – is the intermediate step between the low and high breathing (and so intentionally described last). Let's try to hold in both our abdomen and chest while taking in as much air as possible. It is difficult but not impossible. This is middle breathing.

Full Breath – combines these 3 stages. They follow each other in order: 1, 2, 3. (low, middle, and high).

When you perfect this combined method of breathing, the proper effect should be a wave on your abdomen. It is a wave of harmony (metaphorically speaking), peace and power of a mighty ocean within us.

To sum up:

- we pull in air while pushing out the abdomen
- we then slowly relax solar plexus muscles, allowing the diaphragm to slowly rise
- and finally we push the air up moving the diaphragm as high as possible
- we slowly begin to pull in our belly, then tighten the middle torso – and breathe out
- at the end we pull in our chest puffing out all the air out of the lungs

The rhythm of breathing is very important. So that for example – inhalation takes 6 beats of the pulse (steps, tick of the clock etc) next the full pause takes 3 beats followed by exhalation lasting 6 counts and a 3 count empty phase.

When your reach the count of 16:8:16:8 beats of pulse, without tiring after three full breaths then you've become really good.

Breath control (Sanskrit – pranayama) serves not only to oxygenate your tissues, but also to calm the body and spirit, to calm the mind, and in the end to harmonize all three: body, mind, soul.

<u>Rest and relaxation</u>

Health benefits from practicing meditation are so great that every doctor should prescribe meditation to their patients.

According to the most recent studies by American neurophysiologists the <u>healing process</u> of the body is <u>significantly accelerated</u> when the brain is at a specific state.

The emergence of <u>alpha and theta</u> rhythms in the brain coincides with a marked reduction in the level of stress hormones.

The occurrence of these brain waves significantly increases the efficiency of the <u>immune system</u>. By consciously maintaining the mind in an alpha state, natural healing process occurs much faster and more efficiently.

<u>Ten to twenty minutes</u> a day committed to relaxation is a scientifically proven way of positively improving our Health!

Thus, the enormous benefits of practicing relaxation techniques are the achievement of perfect Health and the elimination of tension and stress related Health problems.

We all know how important it is to be Healthy. Relaxation not only allows us to deal with minor cold and headaches, but also gives us the opportunity to overcome serious diseases – even those called incurable by the doctors.

Relaxation effectively counters the harmful effects psychological and physiological effects of life in a modern world, full of stress and the rush to success.

Relaxation literally gives us a breather. It is a time exclusively for us, where we can delve into ourselves. This time is meant to give our body, mind and soul the strength to wrestle with the problems of everyday life.

The use of appropriate calming techniques can also achieve the ever elusive peace of mind and harmony.

If we take time to relax 2-3 times a day, our body has ample time to regain its inner balance and joy. That in turn allows us to better deal with problems we face in our everyday life, and if those problems are the source of nervous tension their more expedient resolution is a stress preventive measure! In effect taking the time to find our inner balance allows us to handle some problems in such a way that they never even become a stressing factor.

Affirmations, or visualizations used during relaxation result in a better attitude towards self, life and people. This lets us better analyze and solve problems and gives us an opportunity to look at these problems from a distance. All these benefits stand to be gained through regular practice of relaxation.

During the state of deep relaxation and slowed abdominal breathing the body rests.

The state of deep relaxation facilitates healing of the entire body. It slows down metabolism, decreases muscle tension, and the EEG record of brain waves shows that the <u>alpha</u> rhythm appears, a rhythm characteristic of the state of rest and relaxation.

Relaxation activates the right hemisphere of the brain, which makes us more creative, allows us to memorize more information faster, and improves our concentration. We think more creatively and positively.

Top American basketball players benefit from relaxation techniques. This method is used in training Olympic athletes – rowers. Best soccer clubs in Western Europe have in their ranks relaxation and concentration specialists!

What does relaxation provide?

- Speeds up the healing process
- Improves the functioning of the immune system
- Disposes of the negative effects of stress
- Enables us to find our inner balance
- Gives a feeling of tranquility and peace
- Promotes a better attitude toward life
- Improves memory and concentration

Taking time out for relaxation and breathing, often allowed me to survive the difficult hours of severe pain associated with a gout attack.

Alpha waves – electromagnetic oscillations in the frequency range from 8 to 12 Hz – characteristic of a resting human brain, during states of relaxation; occurs when we lie with our eyes closed, usually right before we fall asleep or immediately after waking up. This brain wave frequency is utilized in techniques of fast learning such as the Jose Silva mind control methods.

Beta waves – frequency range of the human brain between 12 and 30 Hz, low amplitude, unsynchronized – the rhythm of preparedness, particularly characterized by normal daily activity, sensory perception and mental work, the specific beta brain activity often accompanies various states after taking certain drugs.

Theta waves – frequency range 4-7 Hz. Theta waves are the most common brain waves. They appear during meditation, trance, hypnosis, intense dreams, and intense emotion. Consciousness at this frequency allows the mind to control physical pain; in extreme cases it can even control bleeding. At this frequency the train of thought becomes fragmented and logical relationships dissolve, which is clearly demonstrated during the thinking process exhibited during dreaming (while we're asleep).

Thanks to the wonderful achievements of modern technology, the work of great musicians, scientists and other people interested in bettering their lives, we have at our disposal enormous wealth of knowledge and excellent, continually improved "tools" available on the market for relatively small cost – all to benefit and improve our health.

One set of such easily available tools are music CD recordings that reflect the above mentioned brain wave frequencies. They are easily available on the internet and can also be purchased in music stores. I highly recommend the purchase and use of such music during relaxation and meditation.

Sleep – a functioning state of the central nervous system, cyclically appearing and passing in a circadian rhythm (daily or 24 hour cycle), during which suspension of consciousness and inactivity of voluntary muscles occur.

The length of sleep in the animal kingdom varies greatly. Giraffes sleep only two hours a day, while bats snooze over 20 hours a day. Some animals (penguins, seals, dolphins) sleep using one hemisphere of the brain at a time. This is characterized by the animal alternately closing one eye by the sleeping hemisphere of the brain. Seals sleep this way, so they can surface and take a breath of air.

Daily sleep requirement in humans is a highly individualized trait. Tests conducted on more than a million participants in California have shown that most people sleep 8 to 9 hour a day, the next largest group sleeps 7 to 8 hours. Throughout his life man sleeps approximately 20 years.

The amount of sleep needed depends on age – a newborn sleeps 18 hours a day, and that amount decreases with age. Newborns and small children divide sleep into several intervals – in adults sleep takes place during one longer part.

The rhythm of falling asleep is regulated by light intensity (the rhythm of sleep/alertness is redefined after long airplane flights) and by social stimuli. In experiments involving complete isolation of people in a room without windows, clocks, television, radio and telephone, subjects given the freedom to choose the moment of falling asleep and waking up, generally operated in the rhythm significantly exceeding thirty hours.

This may mean that a natural rhythm of sleep-alertness is longer than a day – but it is then adjusted to 24 hours.

Evolutionary role of sleep in physiology is not known in precise detail, but due to wide spread presence of sleep in the animal kingdom it is thought to have a fundamental meaning for the nervous system.

There exists a direct correlation between the complexity of the nervous system and the occurrence of sleep. For instance all mammals require sleep. Some hypotheses explaining the need for sleep include:

- saving of energy (decrease in body temperature and energy expenditure)
- hormonal management
- memory consolidation
- stimulation of neurons not activated during wakefulness (to prevent the degradation of the nerves – unused organs atrophy)
- prevention of disappearance of neuronal activity in the locus coeruleus (to prevent any changes in sensitivity – regularly

stimulated organ increases its sensitivity threshold).

Humans require sleep to sustain life and maintain proper mental function. Missing just one night's sleep severely reduces a person's physical and mental ability. Longer sleep deprivation will cause several negative psychological and physiological effects:

- mood swings
- difficulties in concentration
- slowed reaction
- long term (around a week) sleep deprivation or interference with the REM phase can lead to states of psychosis and hallucination, as well as paranoia. REM sleep disorders are often exhibited by alcoholics.
- impaired function of the immune system – abnormal white blood cell count, impaired function of cytotoxic lymphocytes, which normally kill abnormal cells: virally infected or tumor mutated.
- experiments on rats have shown that several weeks of sleep deprivation leads to death.

According to a study conducted at Princeton University in the U.S., it was shown that lack of sleep causes problems in parts of the rat brain responsible for <u>creation of new cells</u>.

Another study published by the Proceedings of the National Academy of Science, showed that in rats, lack of sleep was responsible for a surplus of corticosterone.

Consider all these facts and make a conscious effort to take better care of your sleep.

After gaining full understanding of this chapter and implementing the acquired knowledge and facts, you will make your first step to free yourself from gout pain.

Systematic and conscious control over my actions, allowed me to build a base from which I could continue to completely free myself from gout and its effects – tragic, debilitating attacks of pain.

In the next chapter I discuss the system of proper nutrition in its entirety.

Structure of digestive processes

The human anatomy lessons of primary and secondary education have long been forgotten, by most of us. To refresh our memory, I present brief descriptions of the basic processes of our bodies.

For far too long, have we been looking into the mirror for confirmation of beauty and youth while completely forgetting about the basic needs of the body. Without proper care, our youthfulness and beauty will only be found on old family photographs, and the mirror will become our enemy.

Nutrition – a process of life in which food is provided to every living cell. The delivered food is used by the body as building block material, energy, energy reserve and for regulation.

Is proper eating simply filling your stomach with nutrients?

As it turns out, it is not. Much like during the process of respiration, every cell of our body must be reached by nutrients. From the digested food the organic material in the form of simple nutrients is distributed by blood throughout the body.

Nutrition is vital for every living organism. It is a prerequisite for the maintenance of good health. A diet that is poor in nutrients or exhibits inadequate nutrient absorption and digestion, results in malnutrition and being underweight.

On the other hand eating too often, too much, or eating the wrong foods can cause one to become overweight or obese. Thus Proper nutrition requires the consumption of the appropriate amount of properly prepared food.

Food – nutrients which supply chemical substances important for health and proper development of the organism. These nutrients fulfill many different functions in the body:

- they provide building material for creation, re-building, and maintenance of tissues
- they help to regulate various processes that take place in the body
- they serve as fuel or energy supply

The digestive system – the system of organs which serve to make sure the body is provided with the proper amount of water and nutrients.

The vast majority of nutrients (carbohydrates, fats, proteins) before they are absorbed or assimilated by the body, must first be digested, which involves breaking down of macromolecular organic compounds into simple building block components.

The complex processes of the digestive system can be divided into several correlated and coordinated parts:

- movement of food along the digestive tract (peristalsis)
- digestion (combined with the secretion of digestive juices and bile)
- absorption
- function of the circulatory system (blood circulation, lymph, hepatic portal system)
- coordination of different functions of the digestive system (neural and hormonal regulation with the help of autacoids).

Digestion

The process of digestion involves many mechanisms and systems (hormonal, autonomic nervous system), which in a coordinated manner lead to the breakdown of nutrients into a form that can be absorbed in the gastrointestinal tract.

Mouth

In humans, the digestive process begins immediately after ingestion of food into the mouth. Food ingestion leads to an increase in saliva secretion, which contains the digestive enzyme – salivary amylase. Food is then chewed up and mixed with saliva by the teeth and tongue. Amylase starts digestion of carbohydrates in food. A portion of it then travels through the throat and down the esophagus into the stomach.

Stomach

In the stomach food is mixed with gastric juice, which due to the high concentration of hydrochloric acid inactivates salivary amylase. However, until the acidification of the food, salivary amylase is still active – as a result 20-40% of polysaccharides are broken down.

In the stomach many proteins are digested by pepsin, and gastric lipase initiates the digestion of fats. Not all fats are digested in the stomach due to the lack of emulsification – bile which does digest fats is secreted into the duodenum.

Small intestine

Further digestion of chyme takes place in the small intestine. The partially digested food is transferred from the stomach into the duodenum in batches. Intestinal hormones (secretin, cholecystokinin) stimulate the secretion of bile, intestinal juice, and pancreatic juice. It is here in the small intestine where vast majority of digestion and absorption of food takes place.

The semifluid mass of partly digested food expelled by the stomach into the duodenum is acidic and it is neutralized by the alkaline pancreatic juice, in order to facilitate the action of digestive enzymes such as pancreatic amylase, chymotrypsin, trypsin, lipase, and others.

Bile is secreted into the duodenum which contains bile salts. Its job is to break down emulsified fats, so they become more susceptible to the action of lipase.

Fats are digested by pancreatic lipase, which only works in the aqueous solution, and so only on the surface. As a result of digestion free fatty acids and 2-monoglycerids are formed in the micelles along with bile. In this form they are transported to enterocytes and absorbed.

Besides food absorption small intestines is where the bacterial digestion takes places. Here the undigested food between the fibrils is digested by the intestinal bacteria.

Large intestine

The large intestine is where the absorption of water and a number of vitamins takes place.

Undigested food is excreted as feces during defecation.

Man is considered to be an omnivorous animal because of the ability to digest foods of both animal and plant origin.

Nevertheless, all known cultures categorize foods as those most desirable, those of lesser quality, those to be avoided, and those that are forbidden.

For health reasons it is completely justified to avoid poisonous and those difficult to digest.

All other prohibitions and avoidance are deemed to be assimilated within the socio-cultural framework (religious groups, nations and cultures) and therefore such restrictions vary markedly from one another.

The choice of food in humans is not dictated by instinct as it is in animals. Scientific observations have show that small children up to the age of two, are prepared to put anything in their mouth and eat it, including rocks, beetles, or feces.

The aversion to eating certain things is not innate, but acquired through social interaction. Animals do not exhibit a real emotion of disgust.

Prohibited foods are often associated with the feelings of disgust. The fact that the same food, which in one culture is considered to be non-edible, and can be regarded as a delicacy in another (e.g. dog meat), confirms that the reaction of revulsion is not instinctive – and so it is not related to the properties of the object that generally is biologically edible.

The ability to suppress the reaction of disgust in extreme situations such as famine, and to consume food considered taboo, is individually varied. Usually a very strong aversion in eating causes vomiting, which prefects further consumption.

Most of the known forbidden foods around the world are meat and animal products – only a small number of prohibitions relate to plants. Daniel Fessler and Carlos David Navarrete analyzed 12 cultural groups and found 38 types of food taboos of animal origin, and only 7 foods from plants.

In the world Chinese exhibit the least amount of food taboos – in Europe, the French. Historical data shows that the number of food taboos in Europe has significantly increased in recent times.

Metabolism – the whole of chemical reactions and the associated energy changes occurring in living cells, which forms the basis of all biological phenomena. These processes allow the cell to grow and reproduce, manage its internal structure and respond to external stimuli.

The chemical reactions that make up metabolism are organized into metabolic pathways, in which substrates are most often converted by enzymes in a series of reactions into the final products – metabolites.

Enzymes allow us to carry out thermodynamically less probable reactions, by combining them with other relevant reactions (resulting in the appropriate net thermodynamic or electrochemical effect). They also serve to regulate the speed of reactions in response to changes that take place inside the cell or signals from outside of the cell.

Metabolic pathways can be divided into two broad classes: transforming energy into biologically useful form, and those that supply them with energy so that they may occur.

The first of these are exergonic reactions, during which organic compounds are converted to energy, commonly known as catabolic reactions or more generally as catabolism.

The second require the input of energy, such as the formation of glucose, lipids or proteins, and are called anabolism or anabolic reactions.

Genetically determined metabolic capacity of the organism affects the classification of substances as "useful" or "not useful" (or even "poisonous") and their use and processing. For instance, some prokaryotic organisms (e.g. bacteria of the Beggiatoa genus) use hydrogen sulfide as an energy source, including it in their metabolic pathways; while for animals this is a poisonous gas (H_2S blocks cytochrome oxidase). On the other hand, the metabolic rate determines the amount of food necessary for the proper function of the organism.

Metabolic pathways show a great similarity, even in species with very distant relationship. For example, a set of enzymes, identical in function and similar in structure, involved in the citric acid cycle, can be found in both bacteria Escherichia coli and in complex multi-cellular organisms.

The universality of the metabolic pathways most likely resulted from their high efficiency, and thus a positive evolutionary pressure to maintain them. It also indicated that they've appeared very early in the evolutionary history of life.

Gout Sufferer's Methods and Principles

After applying all the elements of the principles and techniques presented in this chapter, I achieved complete freedom from gout attacks.

The method of drinking water

Only use filtered non-chlorinated water, distilled water or bottled spring water. Mineral water is sold in plastic containers and I dare say that what's written on the label doesn't always correspond to what's in the bottle.

The daily dose of water depends on bodyweight. The rule to follow is this: for every 40 pounds of bodyweight drink one liter of water (4 cups) per day. The water should be consumed in small sips – small but frequent intake of water to better stimulate the smooth function of the liver and kidneys.

Without a constant and proper hydration of the body, there is only a tiny chance of getting rid of the excess uric acid. Remember that well.

This is a critical boundary – insufficient amount of water causes dehydration, and a large amount of toxins and uric acid fail to be removed from the body with urine and feces.

We know how badly toxins interfere with metabolic processes. We also know that toxins are one of the fundamental causes of "aging".

Absolutely do not count other liquids such as coffee, tea, juices or soups, in as your daily intake of water. Very important!

Drink at least ½ a cup of water thirty minutes before meals. Do not drink while eating. You should drink only after the finished meal.

The Morning Routine

The human body requires 90 minutes after waking to completely mobilize processes such as: faster blood circulation, increased heart rate, the processing of stimuli (sight, hearing, touch, smell) requiring large amounts of energy, or brain function. The brain during intense thinking consumes huge amounts of energy, much more than demanding physical work.

How to proceed in the first 90 minutes after waking up?

Here is a ready "routine":

Once you get out of bed and take care of your business in the bathroom, wash your teeth (a large number of microorganisms and toxins accumulated during sleep in the oral cavity, and its better not to eat them), heat some water (in whatever you usually heat it) until it's warm. At the same time in a separate pot of water set up some eucalyptus leaves for inhalation.

You should eat (or drink) one grapefruit or a couple of oranges, while you wait for the water to boil. These fruits stimulate the liver and kidneys perfectly. Their consumption helps to expel left over toxins and uric acid.

Next drink two cups of warm water with freshly squeezed lemon juice. Use a small spoon to do so! (This should take around 15-20 minutes).

While you sip the water a spoon at a time, take breaks to inhale into your nostrils the steam from the pot with eucalyptus. During sleep impurities in your nose and respiratory channels have accumulated. They should be removed because they interfere with free breathing and thus deprive the body of oxygen.

The next step is light physical activity for about 30 minutes. This can be whatever you like to do – yoga, stretching, walking, cycling, swimming, or aerobics – anything.

Your shower should then take about 10-15 minutes – depending on what you're used to.

Now you can turn on your music with the alpha and theta rhythms.

Yesterday you've already decided what you're going to have for breakfast. After the shower you're ready to eat. Take care to make it tasty and make sure it has a lot of vitamins and minerals, whatever you've decided to eat. This is your "foundation" for the day.

Personally, I often drink one or two cups of yogurt with mixed fruits. They are tasty and easy in consumption.

After finishing breakfast, you can spend a few moments reading something motivational or in a prayer. Ten minutes should be enough.

After taking the time to do the above we have created a solid mental and energy base for dealing with problems, surprises and hardships of the day.

Warning: don't bother with anything else in the first minutes of the morning. Do not look up your e-mail, do not review the messages on your voice mail, don't watch television, do not listen to the radio – you do not need any upsetting or destructive information, you have the whole day to take care of that.

The first 90 minutes of the day belong to your mind and body, no one else.

And one more thing – don't worry yourself with something you've "omitted" from the list yesterday, simply do it today with greater care and attention.

Remember – a new habit required 30 days to consolidate. After that it becomes an automatic process. The hardest part in establishing a new habit is the first 10 days.

After ten days have passed – an internal struggle begins – Why am I dong this? What do I need this for? I'd be better of without it... – this is our stubborn self-centered change resistance system (very physical and automatic in operation) responsible for our comfort, dictating its own schedule and discouraging new habits. Do not give up – persevere the next ten days.

The last ten days of the first thirty – a routine starts to establish itself. There is less rebellion, and more and more joy with the results of the new habit.

For the better understanding of the importance of the Morning Routine, I suggest a little Thought Experiment:

Image you've decided to build your dream house. The architect made a beautiful plan for your home. You're happy with the design and visualize yourself in the new, comfortable and functional home.

The construction is started in accordance with the blueprint. You hired construction workers, but you didn't bother to check their recommendations or to see earlier work done by the construction company. Rushed by your impatience to live in your new home you put your trust in them. During the construction of your home, it turned out that the workers laid the foundations improperly. Soon after the first floor was completed; the walls began to crack and bend, and every day, new faults in the construction were being covered up by the dishonest contractor. Inspectors have issued the certificate of occupancy none the less, and deemed your new home as safe and habitable.

After a few weeks you've noticed that something is wrong. Cracks in the ceilings, walls and the appearance of fungus in the basement, totally destroyed the joy you took of living in your new home. Anguish and helplessness descended upon you. Finally you decide to hire an expert/engineer to explain the causes of the problems. Crooked windows and doors have stopped closing.

The engineer determined that the poorly laid foundation was the cause. He said repairs were necessary. You realize that fixing of the foundation won't fix all the broken walls, ceilings, doors and windows. You are now faced with a big overhaul of the entire building.

Think about how easily you could have avoided all the expense, time loss, stress, if you only took the time to check the recommendations and previous work of the construction company or hired a professional to supervise the work.

This is what happens with your body every day. If you fail to lay proper foundations, you can easily imagine later effects.

Fatigue sets in before it's even noon, you lose your concentration, you nervously reply to questions, your irritability makes you quarrelsome and with what little energy you do have left you have to constrain yourself from exploding with anger.

In the evening you spend your free time in front of your TV, glued to the passive "entertainment" because you don't have the energy to undertake any action.

Eventually a number of ailments appear. You become overweight; you feel shortness of breath, aching in your joints sets in, etc.

Life becomes colorless, and you find less and less joy and pleasure in living.

Your body and spirit begin to get sick more often. Doctors and pharmacies are starting to see you as regular client/patient/customer.

Now count all the money spent on doctors, all the days lost at work; add to that all the wrong decisions you've made, because you didn't have enough strength (energy) to better analyze the arguments to be taken into account in the decision process. If you've saved and invested all that you'd probably be a millionaire by now, and we all know how having money makes life easier.

Using the Morning Routine will definitely help you to reach the goals you want to achieve.

Well, we all know the old proverb "you can lead the horse to water, but you can't make it drink".

Your health and your wealth only depend on you Dear Reader. As only you are responsible for your ailments and poverty. Please stop looking around for those responsible, you won't find them. The responsibility for your life rests squarely on your shoulders.

Diet guidelines

You should avoid food products packaged in plastics or Styrofoam when food shopping. No one really knows what chemical reactions occur between a food product and plastic. Keep in line with this rule and there will certainly be health benefits and you won't be having second thoughts.

Avoid heating and cooking in the microwave oven. I have read a lot of articles about the questionable comfort it gives – infrared waves used for heating, can be as damaging as those used for scanning and X-rays.

Is it healthy to get your X-rays every day?

Use dishes made of glass and stainless steel. Dishes made of stone and covered with enamel are also fine.

Get rid of Teflon from your kitchen!

Avoid aluminum – do not wrap your food in aluminum foil. Aluminum easily enters into chemical reactions with food products. The best thing to use is paper, parchment or paper treated with wax, such as the one used to wrap cold cuts at the deli.

Never rush when you eat. You must have ample time to chew your food. Almost 30% of digestion takes place in the mouth – with the use of saliva. I mentioned this in an earlier chapter.

Buy only fresh, good quality, organic products. Each additional dose of synthetic chemicals is an extra chance for a gout sufferer's attack of pain.

Choose all your fruits and vegetables carefully, inspect them to make sure there is no visible damage. You don't know who held the fruit previously and how many "creatures" had the chance to move into the wound.

All fruits without exception must be peeled. The peel is where most of the purines are located, and purines are a known enemy of gout sufferers.

Prepare your food just before meal time. Never prepare your food a day in advance. You won't save much time this way.

Sleep. A good night's rest requires a lot of oxygen in the room where we sleep. Whatever the temperature is outside, always leave at least a small opening in your window. If it is too cold – increase your heating, but never completely close the window.

Keep good care of your bed and mattress. Wash your bed sheets at lease once a week. In a week's time a lot of used up skin and sweat accumulates which is great food for bacteria and mites. Living in symbiosis with them is definitely not worth it.

Determine a regular bedtime hour. An hour before you go to sleep, stop watching movies or television.

The fictional experiences and emotions you witness are taken by our minds seriously – and are not easily distinguished as fiction or reality during sleep. All scenes and phenomena observed right before sleep are taken for "real" and the experienced emotions are treated the same way as actual events.

Emotions always need a lot of time and energy to settle down, so why waste the energy? We don't have an unlimited supply of it.

The body has to relax during sleep and regenerate worn out cells. This process requires energy – and so, simply put – emotions will take away from the energy needed for the body to properly rejuvenate during sleep.

Please do not watch television or movies an hour before bedtime.

During the hour before retiring for the night, it is good to take a short walk, read something light and motivating, and listen to relaxing music. Our mind needs some quiet time after all the experiences of a long and arduous day. The relaxed brain will better supervise the renewal of the body and that is what we sleep for in the first place.

Remember to drink a glass of warm water with freshly squeezed lemon juice a half hour before sleep. This is additional stimulation for important organs – liver and kidneys.

During sleep they work to remove the uric acid. Remember?

<u>Rest and Oxygenation</u> - Work as important part of life as it is, cannot exclude time for recovery. Carefully planning your rest and relaxation is definitely worthy of consideration.

How much time we decide to spend resting and relaxing depends solely on ourselves.

Time does not rule our lives; we can plan how we spend our time.

At least one hour every day should be spent outdoors in communion with nature. It is worth remembering that humans have roamed in open air for millennia: in the forests, mountains and open fields, throughout the entire day.

Our bodies remember those times very well and are not at all happy with being continually locked up in our comfortable "boxes" with artificial cooling, heating and lighting.

A long walk in the woods, or on a beach of a lake or an ocean, cannot be substituted by even the best equipped gym. Outdoor fresh air activity synchronized with the energies of the natural world works miracles for our health.

Especially on a sunny day, such walks activate and facilitate all kinds of positive processes in our bodies.

A brisk walk will give you much more health benefit and relaxation. In the old days when we were still hunter gatherers, many millennia ago, the human body used running only in the times of immediate danger – as a means of escape. Running is not a natural way of moving.

Gout Sufferer's Culinary Art

Culinary art entails all the issues relating to the preparation of dishes. Such terminology is often used to connote the skills of preparing the various dishes in a tasty, nutritious and esthetically pleasing manner.

In different regions of the world, depending on the availability of food, and centuries old traditions, a variety of culinary schools developed.

Some of the basic principles of the Gout Sufferer's Culinary Art:

1. We only use coconut oil for cooking, frying and baking. This is the only oil that the human body is able to digest.
2. We avoid frying our food.
3. We use steaming and boiling.
4. We use fresh butter made from cow milk, as needed.
5. For processing we only use fresh, high quality products of organic origin.
6. We peel the skin of all fruits and vegetables before processing or direct consumption.
7. We don't prepare tomorrow's meal today.

8. For cooking we only use filtered, distilled or mineral water.
9. We only use glassware, porcelain, enamel, stoneware, or stainless steel.
10. We exclusively use sea salt.

Purifying Diet

A few quotes from various sources.

> „For better or for worse, food is the strongest medicine you will ever take"
>
> „Bad diet is not the cause of all diseases, but proper nutrition can cure a lot of them and bring relief in many"
>
> „Eat to live, don't live to eat"
>
> „Some foods are like fire and gunpowder, safe in isolation, but poisonous when combined"
>
> „Change your diet completely, and your mind will change at the same time"

Yes, it isn't said in vain that proverbs are the wisdom of the nations.

First, we must get rid of the „garbage" from our body. In the particular case of gout, the worst junk we need to get rid of are the uric acid crystals, stuck in every tissue of the body – hidden, waiting for the body to have the free resources to remove them.

Oh, these crystals are very patient; sometimes they can lay there for years, waiting to be removed.
It is time to set them free. Here is a purifying diet.

The first thirty days (30 days or 4 weeks) in the process of elimination of uric acid crystal deposits (which have accumulated for years) require special attention and great discipline. In addition to the introduction of new habits (breathing, regular long sleep, drinking water, the morning routine, relaxation) we must get used to a new way of eating.

The new stage of life, life without gout pain, starts with the purchase of the needed food products.

The following is a list of products needed in the kitchen of a gout sufferer. I do not mention quantities, since products need to be replaced on regular basis.

Dairy products: sour cream, buttermilk, plain yogurt, cottage cheese, unsalted butter made from cow's milk, fat-free milk.

Spices: garlic powder, fresh garlic, ginger, cumin, sweet and hot peppers, flax seeds, celery seed, dried parsley, cinnamon, sea salt, clove, rosemary, black pepper, bay leaves, allspice, raisins, thyme, basil, cumin, powdered cumin, nutmeg powder.

Fats: pure coconut oil, fresh unsalted butter.
Fruit: seedless grapes, strawberries, blueberries, raspberry, cherries, plums, pineapple, oranges, lemons, grapefruit, bananas, pears, kiwis, apples, fresh figs, melon, fresh coconut, cantaloupe, watermelon, dates.

Vegetables: brown and red potatoes (not young, and not white), fresh cabbage, celery root and stalks, carrot, parsley (root and leaves), onion, corn on the cob or frozen, avocado, green cucumbers, tomatoes, zucchini, squash.

Grains: brown rice, wild rice, hazelnuts, walnuts, almonds, and other types of nuts, corn.

Sweetening: pure maple syrup, pure (no sugar added) honey, dates, or sweet leaf (stevia).

Now that the shopping is done, and ready products are put away in the fridge and on the shelf; we can start cooking.

During the purifying diet we eat a normal calorie intake (the amount of calories we eat can remain the same as your former diet), we eat a lot of dairy products, especially yogurt – to restore the friendly bacteria flora.

Very important: each day a sufficient amount of calories must be provided, along with vitamins, minerals, proteins (we do not eat meat or fish) and an ample amount of water (40lbs of bodyweight equals 1 liter of water). We cannot lose weight rapidly because each gram of body fat contains the same amount of purines as two grams of muscle. After adhering to all the techniques and methods your body will slowly find its equilibrium bodyweight on its own.

All the recipes are written for a one person meal. Of course if you want to prepare a meal for more people willing to eat from a Gout Sufferer's menu all you have to do is multiply the proportions of ingredients by 2, 3, 4 etc.

Let's Cook!!!

1. Cabbage rolls.

We steam a few detached cabbage leaves in a small amount of water for a few minutes – until they become soft enough to wrap.   After steaming, we wait for them to cool down. The stuffing (see instructions below on how to prepare the stuffing) we then wrap in the cabbage leaves; making rolls (similar to egg rolls in shape, but larger). Thus prepared cabbage rolls we place in a heat resistant stoneware dish and bake for thirty minutes in the oven. After we take the rolls out of the oven, we place them on a plate and pour earlier prepared sauce over them. We place a few slices of fresh pineapple (nothing canned, remember?) and for a side dish we serve a handful of cherries, strawberries or a melon.

Stuffing: Boil a cup of brown rice in two cups of water, until almost tender. We add a spoonful of coconut oil, and some sea salt – for taste, one sweet red pepper sliced into small cubes, one carrot grated into strips, one finely chopped small onion, half a medium peeled and grated apple, one piece of crushed garlic, a handful (tablespoon) of finely chopped parsley.   Grind a few nuts (any kind will do) and 8-10 almonds. Toss all these into the cooked rice and mix it in.

Add a pinch of ground cumin and black pepper for additional flavor.

Sauce for the cabbage roll: peel the skin of two medium-sized tomatoes, and then squeeze the juice into a glass bowl. Mix the squeezed tomato pulp with two tablespoons of yogurt and two tablespoons of sour cream. Flavor with some sea salt and powdered hot pepper, then mix together with the squeezed tomato juice.

2. Celery cutlets.

Take a medium sized celery root and rinse it well, then cook it in a small amount of water, until it becomes soft – but not so soft that is starts to fall apart when slicing it. Thus prepared and slightly cooled celery we peel carefully. Cut the celery into slices about ¾ of an inch thick. We then place the celery slices in hot coconut oil on a frying pen. We toast them until golden brown and turn them over to the other side. Sprinkle with salt and finely chopped fresh rosemary. We place the cutlets on a plate and pour the prepared sauce over them.

On the side we place two tablespoons of cottage cheese, sprinkled with flax seeds and black berries or other fruit (hollow cherries, raspberries, melon or cantaloupe chopped into small pieces, or raisins).

Sauce: We pour two tablespoons of sour cream and two tablespoons of yogurt into a blender. Add a pinch of salt, a pinch of celery seed, two tablespoons of chopped chives or green onions, a garlic clove, a flat teaspoon of fresh butter, a pinch of hot pepper. We blend everything together well... and voila the sauce is ready! Yummy!

3. Potatoes Boiled in „Uniforms" (cooked with the peels).

Take two medium or large brown potatoes (depending on your appetite), wash them well under running water (filtered tap water of course) and boil until tender – prick the potato with a fork to determine if it is ready.

While the potatoes are boiling you can prepare the rest.

Prepare some finely chopped parsley, green onions and dill. You will use this mix to sprinkle the halved potatoes (split in the same matter as fried potato skins, along the longer axis) after first rubbing them with butter. Then add a pinch of salt or black pepper to the ready potatoes.

Prepare a cucumber salad. Place one large thinly sliced green cucumber in a glass, porcelain or stone bowl. Sprinkle with finely chopped chives, a bit of salt and black pepper. A little of green dill won't do any harm. Add two tablespoons full of sour cream – and mix it. The cucumber salad is ready.

Boil a cup of corn kernels (it can be frozen corn). Maize has large amount of protein – and can supply the needed daily doses of easily digestible protein (what's even better – it is purine free).

With this dish serve yourself a piece of melon, an apple or whatever fruit you have a craving for.

Don't forget to drink water after the finished meal. Drink in small sips.

4. Rice with almonds.

Pour into boiling water (two and a half cups of water): a cup of brown rice and half a cup of peeled almonds (almonds are rich in protein).

You can pre soak the almonds in warm water for about an hour – it makes peeling the skin much easier.

Then add a spoonful of coconut oil, two cloves, a pinch of cinnamon, and slat. If you want to make the meal sweeter, add a handful of raisins.

Place two apples in the oven, with peel. After baking the apple, hollow the apple core with a spoon. Pour honey (no sugar added) inside thus prepared apples. Place the apples on a plate and sprinkle them with cinnamon.

Note: do not eat the apple peel! As a side dish prepare one sliced banana and place it next to the apples. Now serve the ready rice with almonds on a plate and ... bon appetite!

5. Corn with cabbage.

First we'll prepare the cabbage. Mince a quarter of a cabbage head into thick chips.

Peel and grate the carrots. Slice or dice a stick of celery into small cubes or slices. Peel a medium sized potato and then dice it into small pieces. Peel one tomato, and then dice it. Prepare one diced medium onion.

Put all the vegetables into a pot with a small amount of water and boil. Let them cook for 5 to 10 minutes. Remove the vegetables and wait for them to cool down, add salt, powdered cumin, medium hot green pepper and mix everything into a mash.

Next, you lace the sliced cabbage into the same pot in which you've cooked the vegetables, and then add a bay leaf with a few grains of allspice. If necessary, add more water (some may have evaporated while you cooked the vegetables) and a flat spoon of coconut oil. Keep the heat low –

do not let the water boil rapidly. Cover the pot and cook for 5-7 minutes, then add the pre-cooked spiced vegetable mix. Cook for another 5 minutes. Once you've finished cooking the cabbage, add chopped parsley and dill. What a great taste!

Cook one cup of corn kernels in lightly salted water.

Grate one juicy, slightly sour peeled apple. Add a tablespoon full of sour cream and mix it. Top the cooked corn with a piece of butter – it will melt on the hot corn. Once the butter melted, cover the corn with the apple and sour cream mix.

Now take the cabbage and serve it on the same plate with the corn. As a side dish – include a quarter of a sliced pineapple.

6. Mashed potatoes with corn. Celery and carrot salad, served with cottage cheese.

Boil two potatoes (medium) until they're soft. After you drain the water from the potatoes, add ½ cup of cooked corn, and some salt (not too much!), a tablespoon of butter and a cup of sweet cream (like that one added to coffee). Mix everything together into a mash. Sprinkle the now ready mashed potatoes with sliced dill and parsley.

Prepare a quarter of a celery root, one garlic clove, one peeled somewhat sour apple, and one carrot. Grate everything into small thin strips. Add a tablespoon of sour cream. Mix. The salad is ready.

Place the mashed potatoes and the salad on a plate; add 2-3 spoons of cottage cheese as an additional source of protein. Your dish is now ready.

7. Potato soup.

One carrot, one parsley root, one red or green pepper, a stick of green celery, one medium size potato, a clove of garlic, one small onion. Wash all the vegetables well under running water, dice them into pieces and throw them into the boiling water. After ten minutes of cooking – remove all the vegetables from the pot, cool them and then mix them.

Add more water to the amount you used to boil the vegetables, so the combined amount of water is about 5 cups. Peel one large potato and dice it into medium sized cubes. Drop the chopped potato and the vegetable mix into boiling water. Add a bay leaf, a few grains of allspice, a pinch of nutmeg, a pinch of salt, black pepper and paprika. Boil for about 15 minutes or until the potato cubes become soft.

8. Tomato soup.

4-5 peeled tomatoes, one medium sized carrot, a stick of green celery, an average size parsley root, half a potato, one onion, a clove of garlic. Dice everything into small pieces and pour into a cup of boiling water. Cook at a lower temperature for about ten minutes. Remove the vegetables and mix them after they've cooled.

Add 4 cups of water to the water you've used to boil the vegetables. Season with a pinch of salt, add chopped basil (or dried) for taste, a pinch of powdered hot pepper, and a tablespoon of coconut oil. Add the vegetables and tomatoes mixed earlier. Cook for about ten minutes.

Put some chopped parsley leaf and basil leaf into a cup of yogurt with sour cream (half a cup of yogurt and half a cup of sour cream) and mix it. Pour the mixture into the pot and boil. After the mix is cooked the soup is finished.

You can serve this soup with a baked potato, salted and buttered.

9. Rice with nectarines.

Pour a cup of brown rice into a pot with three cups of water. Add one tablespoon of coconut oil, add salt for taste, 4 minced dates, a handful of raisins, a teaspoon of honey, half a cup of peeled almonds. Cook the rice for 30 minutes.

Take 4-5 mature fresh nectarines, slice them into four quarters and peel the skin.

Pour sour cream and yogurt into a cup and mix well.

Lay half of the well cooked rice into a glass casserole dish. Place the nectarine slices on top of the rice. Lay the remaining rice of the nectarines. Put the dish in the oven and bake for 25 minutes. Take the dish out of the oven; spread the sour cream yogurt mix over the top of the rice. Put the dish back in the oven for another 10 minutes. The dish is ready.

10. Vegetable soup.

Ingredients: 1 carrot, 1 small onion, 1 parsley root (medium), a stick of green celery, 1/6 of a small cabbage, 1 large red potato. Wash the vegetables under running water (filtered) and dice them.

Pour two liters of water into a pot and boil it. Add a tablespoon of coconut oil, a pinch of salt, black pepper, 1 bay leaf, a few grains of allspice, a pinch of celery seed, powdered hot pepper and cumin.

Drop the chopped cabbage, celery, carrot, onion, parsley into the pot and stir. Cook slowly for 25 minutes. Now add the diced potato. Cook another 10 minutes – until the potato gets soft. Turn the heat off and add a spoonful of sour cream and some chopped parsley leaf.

11. Yogurt with fruits.

Pour a liter of yogurt into a blender. Add slices of peeled mango, 2-3 dates, one peeled kiwi, and a cup of fresh raspberries or blueberries. Use a tablespoon of honey if you need to sweeten the yogurt. Blend everything together. This makes for an excellent first breakfast. Eat half of the fruit yogurt, the other half can wait in the fridge and you'll have it for dessert after dinner.

You can use all the other fruit from the above list to make your own combinations. It's a matter of taste.

12. Rice salad (good for takeout).

Pour 3 cups of water into a pot and boil it. Drop 1 cup of brown rice into boiling water. Add 3-4 diced cloves of garlic, a bit of green celery, a pinch of salt, a spoonful of coconut oil, ½ a cup of diced peeled almonds, and ½ a cup of diced peeled walnuts (or hazelnuts). Let the rice cool after its cooked, and then add one diced peeled apple. Squeeze into it the juice from one fresh onion. Mix well and bon appetite.

13. Corn salad (good for takeout).

Pour a cup of boiled corn in a glass bowl. Dice a ¼ of a pineapple into cubes (of desired size), add 1 sliced banana, 1 sliced kiwi, and mix them into the corn. For better taste; squeeze in some lemon juice. Mix well, and your salad is ready.

14. Potato salad (good for takeout).

Boil 1 large potato. Dice the potato into cubes and put it in a glass bowl. Add an onion (medium size), 2 cloves of garlic, and 1 peeled diced apple. Place everything into the bowl with the cooked diced potato. Add a pinch of salt, celery seeds, marjoram, and black pepper. Squeeze in some fresh lemon juice. Mix everything together, and your salad is ready.

15. Fruit salad with grapes (good for takeout).

Take a banana, a few strawberries, some cherries, a small piece of a cantaloupe, a few fresh fig fruits. Dice them or slice them as you like, and pour into a glass bowl. Add a glassful of seedless grapes. Sprinkle ½ a spoonful of linseed over everything and stir well. Your salad is ready.

Every day of this diet, should include plenty of dairy products, rice and corn.
The diet should be varied and diversified every day, because of the need for the appropriate amounts of vitamins, proteins and minerals.

Once you have completed the purifying diet you can slowly reintroduce other products. But allow yourself only one purine source a day – for instance an egg, or a portion of meat or fish. Use the foods from the purifying diet as the mainstay of your menu. Do not return to your old dietary habits.

Here is a list of products, which should be avoided at all costs:

- yeast and any products that contain yeast,
- alcohol,
- herring,
- sardines,
- snails,
- chicken soup,
- poultry, and poultry offal,
- broth made from meat and bones,
- sausages and all meat cold cuts,
- red meat,
- meat sauces,
- white flour and products made from it,
- asparagus,
- cauliflower,

- fungi,
- dark green vegetables and salads,
- beans,
- peas,
- dried fruits,
- roasted nuts,
- caffeine,
- oatmeal,
- food baked or fried in oils other than coconut oil
- any other fats other than coconut oil
- all synthetic drugs (even small doses of aspirin, unless prescribed by a physician)

The History of My Gout

I examined my life and found a multitude of reasons for the overproduction and deposition of uric acid in my muscles, tendons and bones, which took place many years before the painful attacks of gout began.

Seemingly, one might think that distant past events are not related to gout. This is not the case.

All the diseases you've experienced in your medical history may have a notable impact on the quantity of acid crystallized in your tissues.

Here is the history of events, which most likely had a significant impact on the formation of gout in my organism.

I was born at home in a rural area, without doctor's aid. My mother was assisted by a "midwife". I don't know if she was a real nurse, or self-taught. During my first year as a baby I was sick, and according to my older sister, who to this day likes to bring the subject up, I literally was an unbearable crybaby. I slept little and continually harassed the household with my cries.

I remember a severe pain in my ear, at the age of about four. My grandmother "smoked" my ear, with herbs on a spatula which she heated in a stove. The herbal smoke and the heat of the stove soothed the pain.

At the age of nine or ten, I had a fever and polyps on my tonsils. Diagnosis was – tonsillitis – according to my grandmother. The fever lasted a few days. Besides washing down my throat with salted water, no other cure or medication was used.

In those days few used the doctor's service in cases of ailments so trivial.

My conclusion from the above facts: It is a good thing that I was not exposed to antibiotics or other pharmacological drugs. I avoided the side effects of chemically prepared pharmaceuticals, never fully digested by the human body and probably leaving behind a great deal of difficult to eliminate toxins.

But the most important benefit of these events is the strengthening of my immune system. My organism had to find an antidote for all the bacteria and viruses, and these made the immune system "remember" how to recognize and defeat a threat at the time of attack, thus quickly defeating infections.

To this day, and I'm sixty two years old at this point, I've never had another ear infection or tonsillitis. I've never had seasonal flu. I did not have any fevers, with one exception which I'll explain in a moment.

At twenty years old I had a horrible accident, as a result of which my liver was severed into pieces, and was good for "frying on a pan, without slicing" as one of the operating surgeons jokingly observed.

Additional damage, if I remember correctly, included cracked ribs, bruised spleen, a damaged kidney, and I don't know what else, since frankly I was not interested at all.

What I was interested in, is quick recovery and return to full mobility as soon as possible. A month long stay in the hospital added lung fluid, and other damage, the effect of which in later years made doctors suspect the scarring was of tuberculous origin.

In those days I had boundless confidence in conventional medicine and the people working in the medical field.

I have no idea what drugs were prescribed to me for convalescence, but I am certain they were not the right ones.

After a year of strong bouts of pain, shortness of breath and curling into a ball, with a feldsher's advice, I went to another town to make all the possible laboratory tests, in order to determine the source of the pain.

During the x-rays of my stomach and intestines – and whatever else he was looking at inside my fatigued body – at the moment the doctor touched my duodenum area I lost consciousness. I fainted inside the x-ray machine.

What was the diagnosis? My duodenum was completely scarred by ulcers. The doctor determined that the only possible reason for my duodenal ulcers were the drugs which I kept taking, even though my liver as it turned out has already completely healed.

How much excess acid did my body produce during that time?

Unfortunately, I never sought pleasure in eating. For some strange reason I always treated eating as a necessary evil. For years, I ate only when hungry. In the pursuit of goals I considered important, I simply did not remember about proper nutrition.

After a thorough examination at a clinic where a doctor friend of mine worked, I was given recommendations.

I was not supposed to lose weight; my left kidney was not fully functional. At the moment I lose weight, the kidney drops and stops to function properly.

That's easy to say – don't lose weight.

I took note of the doctor's orders and tried not to lose weight. As soon as I noticed that my clothes fit too loosely, I took it as a warning sign and looked for the reasons of the weight loss.

Of course, I also immediately tried to regain the weight I lost. But that wasn't always easy to achieve.

At the age of thirty-seven, I had another liver operation. This time, they were gallstones, which after the gallbladder was removed during the first operation, grew and accumulated in the bile duct.

The reason for quick gallstone growth was simple: stress, stress, and more stress.

This was a difficult time for me. I was trying to assimilate into the realities of living in a new country. Immigration is always hard.

I was served with another dose of anesthetic – probably a large one, because the operation lasted several hours. At least that is what I was told by the surgeon. And of course another overproduction of uric acid which accumulated in my tissues.

A few years later, I happened to receive anesthesia once again, during a surgery to remove a large ovarian cyst. Every surgery or invasive procedure, takes a toll on the body, so do the drugs associated with it.

In recent years, before the appearance of severe gout pain, personal experiences and events caused me to become depressed, which in turn weakened my will to "take care of myself" and control my food, especially in terms of paying attention to mineral and vitamin content.

Eating large quantities of poultry pâté spread over pastries, because that's what I craved at the time, probably led to the overproduction of uric acid, which the body was not able to properly excrete.

When the attacks did begin to occur, they weren't that acute and I simply suffered them and waited for them to subside. I had not idea why this pain appeared, tortured and disappeared.

Swelling appeared more frequently in the affected areas and lasted longer and longer.

Once diagnosed with gout, I had no idea how to help myself or how to get rid of the pain.

I spent countless hours searching for information on the Internet, information that could help me get rid of gout.

I took a scientific approach to my illness; I began to write down everything in a thick notebook. Systematically, I wrote down descriptions of the attacks, the menu for the day, whether and how I've rested, what stresses I was subjected to and much more information, which started to coalesce into a clear picture of my habits and routines.

By the end of the second year of living with gout, thanks to the extensive notes I've made, I was able to pinpoint the mistakes I've made in my diet, realize that my water consumption was inconsistent, and habitual delaying of rest and relaxation were the primary reasons why I was still suffering from gout. As I've made a conscious effort to correct those areas, my gout diet began to produce results, and the attacks of gout pain became weaker and infrequent.

Through the knowledge of the systems and metabolic processes of the human body, the need for oxygenation by exposure to fresh outdoor air, the "duty" of sleep, rest and relaxation, I created my daily routine.

I now know one more thing, gout thought me to treat my body with humility. I stopped exploiting it mindlessly, and began to respect it.

Conclusion

My sincerest congratulations to you, the Reader!

The fact that you've reached the end of this book demonstrates your total determination to tipping the scales of your life toward "health" (without raising an alcoholic beverage in a toast of course).

You now understand the reasons why you have gout and realize that your liberation from the clutches of gout pain depends exclusively on you.

Consider this sentence: does anyone else's hand force bad, poisonous food into your mouth? The answer is unequivocal – Your Hand does it with the consent of Your Will and by Your Choice.

Theories presented in this book, like the rules and principles of proper nutrition, methods of improving and breathing properly, the need for rest and proper relaxation, the priceless <u>morning routine</u>, the principles of proper and "healthy" cooking, rules for a good night's sleep, ready recipes for gout dishes, all those things are fresh in your memory.

Unfortunately, knowledge alone will not cure you of gout. For you to be healthy again, one more crucial element is required – action.

If the newly acquired knowledge is not applied by you and entered into action, do not expect to be liberated of gout, it is simply impossible.

Start using the new methods and principles beginning today. Keep in mind the principle of thirty days, when applying the lifestyle changes, and you will succeed in making the new diet and all the other methods an effortless habit.

Through persistence, discipline and good will you will certainly regain your health and CONQUER GOUT.

To Your Health!

Teresa Szabo

P.S. I invite you to send any comments about this book, as well as success stories in overcoming gout to this e-mail address:

ts@teresaszabo.com

Appendix

The Morning Routine (90 minutes)

1) After waking up (preferably without an alarm clock) take care of business in the bathroom

2) You set filtered water to boil in a tea kettle and some water with eucalyptus leaf to boil in a pot for inhalation.

3) Go to the bathroom to wash your teeth (during the night a lot of impurities have accumulated in your mouth and it's not advisable to eat them.)

4) You go back to the kitchen and in slow sips you drink 1 to 2 glasses of water with freshly squeezed lemon juice.

5) While slowly drinking your water, in between the small sips, you freely inhale the steam through the nose (steam from the pot with eucalyptus leaf).

6) The next 30 minutes you spend on physical activity: doing gymnastics, cycling, walking outdoors, swimming, practicing yoga, whatever you feel like doing.

7) You take a shower.

8) You prepare and eat breakfast (remember to decide what you'll have for breakfast the night before).

9) After breakfast you meditate or pray.

10) The last 10 minutes of your morning routine you spend reading or watching something motivational.

You are now regenerated, oxygenated, nourished and balanced physically, mentally and psychologically.

You are now ready to face the day's work and responsibilities. Good Luck!

References

Encyclopedia Wikipedia

HealingWell.com

Health Library

H2Ofilters.com

Life Research Universal on Probiotics

Shirley's Wellness Café

Dr. Wallach's "Dead Doctors Doesn't Lie"

Dr. Foster on the Dangers of Prescription Drugs

Dr. Mercola's Total Health

Dr. Balch Prescription for Nutritional Healing

www.ingramcontent.com/pod-product-compliance
Lightning Source LLC
Chambersburg PA
CBHW060415290526
45791CB00002B/761